Prologue to Change:

African Americans in Medicine in the Civil War Era

By

Robert G. Slawson, MD, FACR

The NMCWM Press

© Copyright 2006 by Robert G. Slawson, MD, FACR

All rights reserved. No part of this book may be used or reproduced without written permission of the author and the publisher, except in the case of brief quotations embodied in critical essays and reviews.

Published by: The NMCWM Press
The National Museum of Civil War Medicine, Inc.
P.O. Box 470
Frederick, MD 21705
Phone: 1-800-564-1864
Museum Store Phone: 1-301-695-5225
Fax: 1-301-695-6823
www.civilwarmed.org
email: museum@civilwarmed.org

ISBN# 0-9712233-4-3

The NMCWM is a not-for-profit 501(c)(3) corporation

Book design by: Scott Edie, E Graphics, Brunswick, MD

Printed by: Signature Printing, Gaithersburg, MD

Printed and bound in the United States of America

First Edition

Cover Illustration: Howard Medical College Faculty, 1869-1870. Alexander T. Augusta (front row, far left) and Charles B. Purvis (front row, second from right) were the only two African Americans on the faculty at that time. *Used by permission of the Moorland-Springarn Research Center, Howard University, Washington, D.C.*

Table of Contents

Acknowledgements		v
Foreword	Carl W. Mansfield, MD, FACR, FACNM	vii
Chapter 1:	Introduction	1
Chapter 2:	The Beginnings	4
Chapter 3:	The Nineteenth Century	7
Chapter 4:	Known Medical School Graduates	9
Chapter 5:	Possible Medical School Graduates	19
Chapter 6:	Physicians Without Degrees	21
Chapter 7:	Union Army Physicians	27
Chapter 8:	Commissioned Officers	30
Chapter 9:	Contract Surgeons	35
Chapter 10:	Conclusion	42
Bibliography		43
Index		48

Dedication
and
Acknowledgements

This book is dedicated to the pioneers who are the subjects of this report. Their actions at that time and place were against all odds. Their individual and collective successes need to be remembered, and they must be given their place as forerunners of the modern world.

In addition to those whose actions are described here, I need to thank many people who encouraged this effort. This long list starts with Larry Denney and Dalyce Newby and includes my wife, Mavis, and the staff of the National Museum of Civil War Medicine as well as Carl Mansfield, a long-time friend and former boss. I owe thanks to people such as Terry Hambrecht, Margaret Humphreys, Peter D'Onofrio and Terry Reimer who have helped the project grow. Terry Reimer has been tireless in her editorial assistance. I particularly thank the many helpful librarians and archivists who made this task so much easier. There are many others whom I bored with my enthusiasm. I thank one and all!

Foreword

The Civil War was a defining moment in the history of the United States. Only recently, the role of African Americans in that war has come to light. This book recounts some of the contributions made by them as medical officers. Little is known about them since some were not even listed as part of the Army Medical Corps.

Dr. Robert Slawson is a Master Docent at the National Museum of Civil War Medicine in Frederick, Maryland. He has extensive knowledge of Civil War history and the medical aspects of that tragic but inevitable conflict.

Dr. Slawson has chosen a difficult subject to write about because of the lack of documentation. All forms of "media," books, papers, and official records would probably not have commented on the life and actions of these slaves or Freedmen. From the historical review, other than being a slave or Freedman, the African American was invisible. Their daily life, struggles, joys, failures and accomplishments were not recorded. No one was interested. Usually during that time, African Americans were noticed or written about only for comedy or ridicule. On the positive side, this work illustrates the resiliency, determination and refusal to be "held back" that these men exhibited.

With this in mind, it is even more remarkable that Dr. Slawson was able to glean bits of information from historical writings. He has created for us a small picture, a window into the past, to illustrate that these were individuals who in the face of an oppressive society and against overwhelming odds and restrictions made personal accomplishments and contributions to this society.

It should be noted that there were whites at that time who were fighting against slavery, teaching, and assisting freed and bound men and women to attain a better life.

This is the first documented evidence of a segment of American history. It is a thorough review of the available information. There is much about this period and the actions and accomplishments of the African American physicians that is unknown. It is hoped that this book will encourage the presentation or submission of more information about a remarkable people who lived and struggled during these times.

Carl W. Mansfield, MD, FACR, FACNM

Chapter 1

Introduction

Histories of medicine and of medical education often have been written with little regard for the social and political changes occurring at the time. Traditionally, many aspects of medicine have been ignored.[1, 2] An example is the rise of the objections to the prevalent medical philosophy regarding the origin of disease and of its treatment. Because of the impact these changes had on medicine, historians have provided supplemental information concerning this tumultuous time.[3]

Traditional medicine was dominated by white males and centered on the concept of humors and the balance of the systems of the body. Treatment was given with the intent of causing severe symptoms opposite from those of the disease. This was, of course, in the time before the recognition of bacteria as the cause of many diseases. Such treatment often led to strong physical reactions in the patient, and early in the nineteenth century public sentiment arose against the severe discomfort caused by heroic medicine with its reliance on heavy metals. Many traditional physicians began withholding some of these agents and promulgating a more natural approach to patient care. Other practitioners started promoting alternative treatments, and by the second quarter of the nineteenth century began opening medical schools that taught the use of these alternatives.

Samuel Thomson was a self-taught herbalist who marketed a system of botanic medicine using only vegetable sources. This system became known as Thomsonian medicine. Gradually this evolved through "reformed" medicine into a middle-of-the-road approach called "eclectic" medicine. Samuel C. F. Hahneman in Germany promoted the use of very small doses of medicine that in larger doses would have caused the same symptoms as the disease being treated. This system was called "homeopathy" because it caused few symptoms in the patient. The homeopathic physicians called traditional medicine "allopathy" because of the treatment-induced changes in the patient. These divisions in medical philosophy were called "sects," and the non-traditional sects were known as "sectarian" medicine. By the time of the Civil War, sectarians constituted about ten percent of all physicians in America and schools of Thomsonian medicine, eclectic medicine, and homeopathic medicine had been opened throughout the country. It must be noted that the sectarian schools as a group were more liberal than the traditional medical schools and enrolled larger numbers of women and African Americans as students.

The entrance of women into formal medical education and the medical profession stimulated a large body of literature. Interestingly, the community at large was more willing to contribute financial aid to help women establish medical schools than had been the case in the establishment of traditional medical schools. The social struggles and ramifications caused by this advance are well-documented and reported.[4-8]

Traditional histories are strangely silent, however, about another potential social upheaval—the appearance of African American medical practitioners. It is true that initially only small numbers were involved and the social implications seem to have been generally ignored. The first African American medical school graduate did not appear until 1837.[9] From the early years, African Americans practiced traditional medicine that was learned in the traditional way, by apprenticeship, as well as using the herbal and folk medicines that came with them from Africa.[9, 10]

Early medical care in this country began with very few school-trained practitioners. Because of the scarcity of trained physicians, most care was given by persons without formal training. Although in Europe the title "doctor" was restricted to a small group of elite college and medical school graduates, from the beginning in America all care-givers appropriated the title without regard to training. As the population grew, so did the need for care-givers with medical training. The early informal practice of learning on-the-job by assisting a trained practitioner was replaced by a formal apprenticeship with signed articles of indenture. Responsibilities of the preceptor and of the student were detailed. Those with the financial capability often followed this training with a trip to Europe to attend or even to graduate from medical school. In the last half of the eighteenth century, medical schools were started in this country to provide formal didactic lectures to supplement the clinical training of the apprenticeship.

John Morgan founded America's first medical school in 1765, the Philadelphia College of Medicine, now the University of Pennsylvania College of Medicine, in Philadelphia, Pennsylvania. Several schools followed using the same format, with four to six professors who owned the school and lectured in the various medical subjects thought to be important at the time. A "year" of classes lasted three to four months and the same lectures were repeated the next year. To graduate, a student had to complete at least three years of apprenticeship and two years of lectures. Gradually the schools in the larger cities provided clinical training to replace the outside apprenticeship. Students who had the interest and the financial means still followed graduation with a trip to Europe for further training and experience. In the first quarter of the nineteenth century, at least 80 percent of all doctors entered practice with an apprenticeship only. By 1860 this had changed so that 80 percent of practitioners in America were medical school graduates.

Unfortunately, there is very limited documentation about African Americans and their entry into formal medical education. This lack of comment in the lay press and medical literature of the time suggests that the community at large did not feel threatened by the advance of these few African Americans into the medical arena. The medical public and press had reacted strongly to the rise of sectarian medicine[1] and to the entrance of women into this exclusively male province.[4] In any event, there is little written record of the early movement of African Americans into medicine in the United States,[11, 12] although several of the early African Americans have been the subjects of biographies recording the undoubted contributions they made. Many books and articles written in the late twentieth century have added little to this epoch and some have even ignored it completely.[13-15] The appearance of African Americans in medical practice in this country prior to the end of the Civil War and emancipation certainly was significant.

Several aspects of this increasing involvement of African Americans in mainstream American medicine will be addressed. This covers the early years of America as well as the move to the more formalized world that existed by the time the Civil War began. The various African American practitioners and the different routes taken to enter medical practice provide fascinating stories of courage and determination. Of course, the primary incentive for this work relates to those African Americans who served with the Union Army during the Civil War.

Chapter 2

The Beginnings

The majority of early African American physicians were slaves who practiced medicine among their people. However, the first documented African American physician in America, Lucas Santomé, was free (Table 1). He had been trained in Holland and practiced in New Amsterdam.[10] In 1667 he was rewarded for his services to the colony with a grant of land in New Amsterdam. He practiced there under Dutch rule and later under British rule. Further biographical data on Santomé is not available.

The first documented incident of preventive medicine practiced in the United States can be credited to a slave in Massachusetts.[10] In 1706 Cotton Mather, a Puritan Congregational minister, acquired a slave called Onesimis who had been brought directly from Africa. Because the city of Boston was concerned about smallpox, Mather asked Onesimis whether he had had this disease. Onesimis responded that he was given an operation to prevent it and showed the scar to Mather. Onesimis described the process used in Africa to stay free of smallpox, by those brave enough to have it done. A small cut was made in the skin of the arm and scrapings from a smallpox sore from another person were inserted. As a result smallpox occurred in the person inoculated, but it was usually very mild. In a letter dated 1716, Mather conveyed this information to John Woodward of the Royal Society in England[10] and also to his friend, Dr. Zabdiel Boylston in Boston. Boylston subsequently inoculated several people, including his own six-year old son.

Table 1: Early Practitioners

Seventeenth Century	*Location*
Santomé, Lucas	New Amsterdam/New York

Eighteenth Century	
Onesimis	Massachusetts
Simon	Philadelphia
Runaway	South Carolina
Primus	Connecticut
Caesar	South Carolina
Derham (Durham), James	Philadelphia & New Orleans

There was tremendous public reaction against this procedure. In the New England smallpox epidemic of 1721-1722, there were 844 deaths among 1,500 cases of smallpox. Boylston, and a few others, had inoculated 286 people and only 6 of these died. King George I and the Royal Society subsequently honored Boylston, who never publicized the true source of his information,[10] although one history of public health does credit an unnamed slave as providing the information to Mather.[16] As early as 1714, smallpox inoculation had been discussed in the *Transactions of the Royal Philosophical Society* as being practiced in Greece and Turkey. The first use of inoculation in England after 1721 was at the behest of Lady Mary Wortley, wife of the British Ambassador to Turkey.[16] Vaccination, the use of pus from the cowpox virus (vaccinia) as opposed to the smallpox virus (variola), was introduced in England by Edward Jenner in 1796.[16]

Other slaves were credited with knowledge of medicine. In 1740 the *Pennsylvania Gazette* in Philadelphia carried an advertisement for a runaway slave called Simon, describing him as "able to bleed and draw teeth, pretending to be a great doctor among his people."[9] A similar notice in the Charleston, South Carolina, *City Gazette and Daily Advertiser* in 1797 declared of a fugitive slave (no name given) "He passes for a doctor among his people and it is supposed practices in that capacity about the town."[9] No other information has surfaced on either of the gentlemen.

In 1740 mention is made of a slave named Primus owned by Dr. Alexander Wolcott of the Wolcotts of Yale in Windsor, Connecticut. He apparently worked with Wolcott for several years and, as a reward for his services, Primus was given his freedom. He established a practice in Windsor where he worked for many years while maintaining a cordial relationship with Dr. Wolcott and the other physicians of the town.[9]

The Charleston, South Carolina, *City Gazette and Daily Advertiser* of May 9, 1750,[10] stated that a slave named Caesar was given his freedom after the General Assembly of South Carolina voted funds for this purpose as well as an annual stipend of 100 pounds. This was a reward for a cure that he had developed for rattlesnake bite.[17] This "cure" contained such items as horehound, sassafras, wood ashes, and tobacco. He also had an article published in *Massachusetts Magazine* in 1792 describing a cure for poison, and in 1799 Buchan's *Domestic Medicine* listed his cure.[17] No other details of his life are known.

The first African American physician known to be trained by the traditional medical practice of the time, by apprenticeship, was James Derham (also spelled Durham).[9, 10, 17] Derham, born a slave in Philadelphia, Pennsylvania, grew up in the house of Dr. John Kearsley, Jr., one of the founders of the Philadelphia Medical Society. Derham started his medical apprenticeship under Kearsley. On the death of Kearsley, he was sold to and assisted Dr. George West, a surgeon in the British Sixteenth Regiment in the

Revolutionary War. At the end of the war, Derham was sold to Dr. Robert Dove, a physician in New Orleans, Louisiana. Because of Derham's medical ability and service, Dove liberated him on "easy" terms, which are not described. After obtaining his freedom, Derham developed a successful medical practice in New Orleans.

These vignettes from the seventeenth and eighteenth century provide insight into the potential role this group of people would play in the future. These African Americans contributed significantly against all odds. With the increased growth of formal education in medicine in America, it is necessary to acknowledge the challenges and accomplishments of these pioneers.

Chapter 3

The Nineteenth Century

For the nineteenth century, more information is available and more African American physicians can be identified. However, many are known only by name with little or no biographical information available—dates of birth and death are often not reported and details of their medical training are not always known. But this period does introduce the first African Americans with medical degrees, some obtained outside the United States. In addition, a significant number began to practice with only an apprenticeship, as was also true of the white population at the beginning of the century. The percentage of all physicians with medical degrees gradually increased during this period, and this is also true of the African American doctors.

The physicians identified from this period can be separated into several groups. The first are those known to have been granted medical degrees from known schools. As far as possible, issuance of these degrees has been verified from the appropriate medical school archives. Morais,[17] in his book *The History of the Negro in Medicine*, states that the professionally-schooled African American physicians were far fewer in number than those practicing by apprenticeship, as had been true for European Americans earlier in the nineteenth century. Yet he, as did others writing of this period, lists far more medical school graduates than apprentice physicians. It is possible that this shows that a medical diploma represents a more formal education, and therefore greater status in the community.

The second group is doctors mentioned as having been graduated from a medical school but the school was not specifically identified. To date no medical school has been identified for some of these individuals. A subgroup of graduates includes physicians who subsequently served in the Union Army during the Civil War, and therefore a medical degree might be presumed.

Instances were found where men were said to have been graduated from a certain medical school, but the archives of that school show no record of attendance or only a record of attendance with no graduation.[9-11] In some cases further searching has revealed graduation at a school different than reported. In one instance, a physician was listed in one report as having been graduated from a certain school[18] but another report listed a different school,[9] while neither school today has any record of attendance for the man. Medical school names during this period were often confused, and many schools were referred to in ways that were different from their proper names. Several of the graduates were from schools of branches, or sects, of medicine that no longer exist, and due to the closure of these schools, the location of any existing archives is unknown. Many traditional medical schools closed and were merged with existing schools, so archives can often be traced and searched. Some schools closed without mergers, however, and their archives have not been found. In general this is true of the sectarian schools, and it has frustrated the efforts of documenting the graduation of students from those schools. A further complication in tracking students is the fact that it was common for students to attend more than one medical school prior to obtaining a diploma. This was done, in part, because schools repeated the same lecture schedule each year. Rotation to different schools gave more variety to the information received.

As a group, African American physicians of this period, with or without a degree, were more educated than most of their African American peers, and the majority of them were actively involved in abolitionist and anti-slavery activities. By separating these physicians into groups according to the route taken for entry into medical practice, it is easier to understand the dynamics of the events as a whole.

Chapter 4

Known Medical School Graduates

By the end of the Civil War, there were twenty-three known African American medical graduates. The first African American man to receive a medical degree, although it was obtained outside the United States, was James McCune Smith (Table 2).[9, 10] Smith was born in 1811 of free parents in New York City, where his father was a prosperous merchant. He attended the African Free School and subsequently decided to study medicine. When he was unable to gain admittance to a medical school in the United States, Smith went to Scotland where he was admitted to the University of Glasgow. Following the educational requirements in Scotland, he received a Bachelor of Arts degree in 1835, a Master of Arts degree in 1836, and finally his Doctor of Medicine degree in 1837.[19] After graduation he returned to New York, established a successful practice and opened two apothecary shops. For many years he was a physician to the Colored Orphan Asylum in New York City which had opened a hospital in 1836, and was the only African American officer of that institution.[9] As with most educated free African Americans of the time, he became a spokesman for the abolition movement [17] and had at least two letters publicly printed.[20] Smith died in 1865 of a heart attack at age 54.

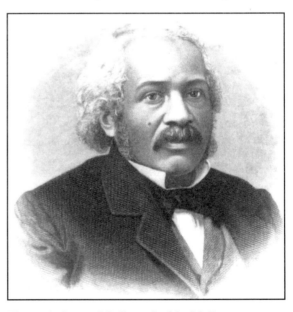

Figure 1. James McCune Smith, M. D.
Dr. Smith was graduated from the University of Glasgow School of Medicine, Glasgow, Scotland, in 1837, thus becoming the first African American to receive a medical degree. *Used by permission of Source Prints & Photographs/Moorland-Spingarn Research Center, Howard University, Washington, D.C.*

David James Peck was graduated from Rush Medical College in Chicago, Illinois, in 1847,[21] and was the first

Table 2: Known Medical School Graduates

Name	School	Location	Year	
Smith, James McCune	University of Glasgow	Glasgow, Scotland	1837	X
Peck, David James	Rush Medical College	Chicago, IL	1847	X
DeGrasse, John Van Surly	Medical School of Maine	Brunswick, ME	1849	X
White, Thomas Joiner	Medical School of Maine	Brunswick, ME	1849	X
Ray, Peter William	Castleton Medical College	Castleton, VT	1850	W
Bias, James Joshua Gould	Eclectic Medical College	Philadelphia, PA	1852	S
Rock, John Sweat	American College of Medicine	Philadelphia, PA	1852	S
Dunbar, Charles	Medical Department of Dartmouth College	Hanover, NH	1853	X
Laing, Jr., Daniel	Medical Department of Dartmouth College	Hanover, NH	1854	X
McCord, David O.	Medical College of Ohio	Cincinnati, OH	1854	C
Taylor, William Henry	National Medical College	Washington, DC	1856	X
Creed, Cortlandt van Rensselaer	Yale University	New Haven, CT	1857	X
Roudanez, Louis Charles	Medical Department of Dartmouth College	Hanover, NH	1857	X
Watson, Samuel C.	Western College of Homeopathy	Cleveland, OH	1857	X
Ellis, William B.	Medical Department of Dartmouth College	Hanover, NH	1858	X
Leach, Robert B.	Western College of Homeopathy	Cleveland, OH	1858	X
Augusta, Alexander Thomas	University of Toronto	Toronto, Ontario	1860	X
Rapier, Jr., John	Iowa College of Physicians and Surgeons	Keokuk, IA	1863	N
Boseman, Benjamin A.	Medical School of Maine	Brunswick, ME	1864	X
Lee (Crumpler), Rebecca	New England Female Medical College	Boston, MA	1864	X
Purvis, Charles Burleigh	Medical Department of Western Reserve College	Cleveland, OH	1865	X
Tucker, Alpheus W.	Iowa College of Physicians and Surgeons	Keokuk, IA	1865	G
Abbott, Anderson Ruffin	Toronto School of Medicine	Toronto, Ontario	1867	X

X – Checked by Author (See text)
N - Checked by Newby (See Bibliography)
W- See Waite in Bibliography
C – See Chew in Bibliography
G – See "Genealogy Records.." in Bibliography
S – Archives of these sectarian schools cannot be found

African American to receive a diploma from a medical school in the United States.[9, 10] Peck practiced unsuccessfully in Philadelphia for two years, then left in 1850 to go to California. On the way he met Dr. Martin Delany, a boyhood friend from Pittsburgh, Pennsylvania, and became involved in Delany's emigration movement to Nicaragua. This attempt to establish a colony for African Americans outside the United States failed in 1855, as did most such efforts. Although Delany returned to the United States, Peck stayed behind in Nicaragua to practice medicine, apparently never returning to the United States.

The next two men to receive medical degrees were graduated from the Medical School of Maine, affiliated with Bowdoin College, in Brunswick, Maine, in 1849.[9] They were John Van Surly DeGrasse[22] and Thomas Joiner White.[22] No additional information is currently available on White except for the fact of his graduation in the same class as DeGrasse.

Because diplomas were awarded alphabetically, DeGrasse was the second African American to receive a medical diploma in the United States when he was graduated in 1849. Following graduation he studied in Paris for two years, working with Dr. Alfred Velpeau. He returned to New York where he practiced for only a short time before moving to Boston, Massachusetts, where he achieved a successful practice and became a member of the Massachusetts Medical Society. In 1863, after the creation of the United States Colored Troops, he obtained a commission as an assistant surgeon and served in South Carolina with his regiment. After leaving the military service he returned to his practice in Boston.

Peter William Ray was born in 1823 and was graduated from Castleton Medical College in Castleton, Vermont in 1850.[23]

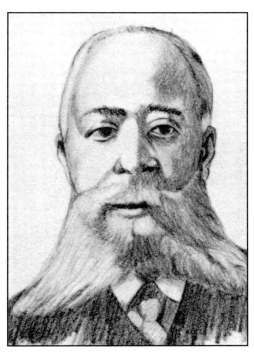

Figure 2. Peter William Ray, M.D. Acting Assistant Surgeon, United States Colored Troops

Dr. Ray was a graduate of Castleton Medical College, Castleton, Vermont. He had an extensive practice in New York and operated several pharmacies. *Used by permission of the Association for the Study of African American Life and History.*

He had been apprenticed to Dr. James McCune Smith in New York, and then attended one year of classes at the Medical School of Maine.[22] Ray then transferred to Castleton where he received his medical degree. After graduation, he returned to his home in Brooklyn, New York, where he opened a drug store and established a large, successful practice, particularly among the German immigrants. Ray developed a good reputation in the treatment of diseases of children and in obstetrics. He was active in local medical circles and a member of the New York State Medical Society. One year he was a delegate to the New York State Medical Association meeting in Canada. He practiced in Brooklyn for more that fifty years.[9, 11]

The next known graduates were in 1852. The "well esteemed" Dr. James Joshua Gould Bias[17] was graduated from the Eclectic Medical College of Philadelphia. This was a non-traditional school, and no record of the fate of its archives has been found. Bias practiced medicine in Philadelphia and was a practical phrenologist. A phrenologist studies the contours and convexities of the head and assigns personality and character traits to the individual accordingly, and then recommends treatment and a course of action. He was also very active in the abolition movement, and his home and office were important to the Underground Railroad. Bias died in 1860 in Philadelphia.

Dr. John Sweat Rock is better known,[9, 10, 17] although more for his actions in the abolition movement and in law than in medicine. He was freeborn in 1825 in Salem, New Jersey, where he attended public school and subsequently became a teacher.[24] He apprenticed in medicine with two white physicians, Quinton Gibbons and Jacob Sharpe, and then applied to medical school. After his application was rejected, he apprenticed in dentistry with

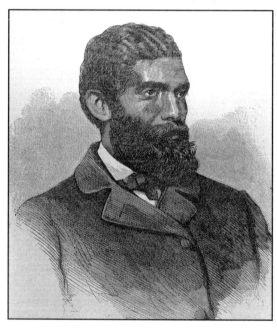

Figure 3. John Sweat Rock, M.D.
Dr. Rock was a graduate of The American College of Medicine in Philadelphia. He also became a lawyer and a member of the Massachusetts Bar. He was the first African American to be allowed to argue cases before the Supreme Court of the United States. *Used by permission of the Boston Athenaeum.*

Dr. Samuel Harbert in New Jersey. He was certified in dentistry in 1849 and opened a dental practice in Philadelphia in 1850. He later decided to try medical school again and was admitted to the eclectic school, the American College of Medicine in Philadelphia, Pennsylvania, and was graduated in 1852. That same year he also married Catherine Bowers from Philadelphia. Rock initially practiced both medicine and dentistry in Philadelphia, then moved to Boston, Massachusetts, in 1853, opening an office at 83 Phillips Street. During the 1850s he became very prominent in abolition activities, as did many of the educated African Americans of the time. He was a featured speaker at the 1858 Annual Crispus Attucks Celebration in Boston and stated "Black is beautiful," although this statement would not be recalled for many years. It is known that Harriet Tubman stayed in his home in Boston on several occasions.[25]

When Rock became ill from an unstated medical problem, he decided to go to Paris for medical treatment. A controversy arose about his passport because African Americans were not considered citizens and were not eligible for passports. Ultimately, with the influence of Senator Charles Sumner, Massachusetts passed a law allowing passports for African Americans, and Rock went to Paris. He was told by physicians in Paris that his health was not good enough to continue practicing medicine so upon returning to Boston in 1859, he closed his medical-dental practice. In 1860 he studied law by apprenticeship, and in 1861 he was admitted to the Massachusetts Bar and opened a law office at 6 Tremont Street in Boston. Sometime in the next few years he was appointed a Justice of the Peace by Governor John A. Andrew. He worked as a recruiter for the 54th and 55th Massachusetts Infantry Regiments, after Colored Troops were finally authorized in 1863.

Rock became the first African American allowed to argue cases before the Supreme Court of the United States,[17, 26] having been presented on February 1, 1865, by Senator Charles Sumner from Massachusetts and accepted by Chief Justice Salmon P. Chase.[20] It should be noted that while sources state Rock was graduated in 1852 from the American College of Medicine in Philadelphia, other sources say that this school had one class in 1853-1854, closed until 1856, reopened and then closed again after graduation in 1861.[3] Rock's graduation date, then, is in question and may have been 1854. As with so many other non-traditional schools, the archives have vanished. Rock was also active in abolitionist circles and several of his speeches and letters have been published.[20] Rock died in 1866.

The Medical Department of Dartmouth College in Hanover, New Hampshire, provided the next two known graduates, Charles Dunbar of New York City in 1853[27] and Daniel Laing, Jr., of Boston in 1854.[27] Little is known about the life of Dr. Dunbar except that he was from New York City and that his medical graduation was confirmed from the archives at Dartmouth.

Laing, along with the African Americans Martin R. Delany and Isaac Snowden, was admitted to Harvard Medical School in the fall of 1850.[9] For that same session, Harvard also admitted a woman, Harriot Kesia Hunt.[7, 28] The affluent students of this school in liberal New England rebelled[1] since they did not want to go to school with a woman or with African Americans. Dr. Oliver Wendell Holmes, Dean of the Harvard Medical School at that time, bowed to the pressure from the students and from his Board of Trustees and told the four students that they could only stay to the end of the session. Miss Hunt resigned immediately and Delany apparently stayed until the end of the session. It is unclear from the existing descriptions when the other two men left. These two were sponsored by the American Colonization Society and had agreed to emigrate to Africa after receiving medical degrees.[29] Laing is the only one of the group who is known to have received a subsequent medical diploma, in 1854, but it is not known whether he actually emigrated, as was his original intent.

David O. McCord also was graduated in 1854, from the Medical College of Ohio in Cincinnati.[30] McCord was freeborn in Kentucky in 1830 and his family moved to Illinois in 1833. He apprenticed in medicine and then attended medical school. Following graduation in 1854, he established a practice in York, Illinois. In 1862 he was commissioned assistant surgeon with the 66th Illinois Infantry but spent his time on detached duty serving at a Freedmen's hospital. In December 1863, he was promoted to surgeon, equivalent to a major, and was appointed as Medical Director and Inspector of Freedmen in the Department of Tennessee and the State of Arkansas. His orders describe him as "of African descent" although his original commission was in a white unit and was prior to the creation of the United States Colored Troops. After the war, he returned to his practice in Illinois and, at the time of his death in 1874, he was a member of the Illinois chapter of the American Medical Association.

William Henry Taylor was graduated from the National Medical College in Washington, D.C., in 1856.[31] This graduation was of particular significance because the National Medical College, now George Washington University, was the first medical school south of the Mason-Dixon Line to grant a medical degree to an African American. The only other school with known attendance of an African American was Washington Medical College in Baltimore. The National Medical College's alumni records state that Taylor died in 1889, but no other history is known about him.

In 1857 there were three more African American medical graduates: Cortlandt van Rensselaer Creed, Louis Charles Roudanez, and Samuel C. Watson, adding Yale University in New Haven, Connecticut, to the list of schools allowing African American student attendance.

Creed was freeborn in 1835 in New Haven, Connecticut. He was graduated from the Medical School of Yale University in 1857[32, 33] and was the first African American to be graduated from that medical school. Following graduation, he developed a successful practice in New Haven. Creed had been an early advocate for the use of African American troops in the Union Army. In 1863 he obtained an appointment as acting assistant surgeon with a Connecticut regiment and served with his regiment during the war. After the war, he returned to his practice in New Haven. Creed died in 1900.

Louis Charles Roudanez[34] was freeborn in 1823 in New Orleans, Louisiana. He initially studied in Paris, receiving a medical degree from the University of Paris in 1853. He returned to the United States and obtained a second medical degree from the Medical Department of Dartmouth College in 1857,[27] practicing in New Orleans where a sizable enclave of freeborn African Americans lived. He and his brother, Jean-Baptiste, published newspapers from 1862 to 1868 and advocated equal civil rights for African Americans. The extent of other abolitionist activities by Roudanez is unclear. His brother, with a group of freeborn African Americans from Louisiana, wrote and delivered to President Lincoln a resolution and proposal for African American suffrage in the newly-constituted Union government in Union-occupied Louisiana.[20] Roudanez died in 1890.

Samuel C. Watson was graduated in 1857 from the Western College of Homeopathy, a sectarian school in Cleveland, Ohio, whose records of medical graduates surprisingly have been preserved.[13] He was the first African American graduate of a school of homeopathy in the United States.[35] Watson practiced for a short time in Ontario, Canada, where a large community of freeborn and former-slave African Americans lived, and then went to the gold fields in British Columbia in the early 1860s. He moved to Detroit in 1863 and, according to family history,[13] was never allowed to practice medicine. Because of this, he established a prescription drug store that became one of the most successful in the city. Dr. Watson became involved in local politics as well, and in 1884 he was a delegate to the Republican National Convention, the first African American to fill this position.

William B. Ellis was graduated from the Medical Department of Dartmouth College in 1858.[27] Also in 1858, the second African American graduate from the Western College of Homeopathy in Cleveland, Ohio,[35] was Robert B. Leach[17] of Philadelphia. Unfortunately, no other biographical information on Leach was found.

Ellis is reported to have served as a physician with the Army during the war. Unfortunately, few details of his life before and after his medical graduation are known, except that he received an appointment as an acting assistant surgeon in March 1864, serving in Washington, D.C.

Alexander Thomas Augusta[36] was freeborn in 1825 in Norfolk, Virginia, and although it was illegal in that area, he was taught to read and write as a child. He decided to become a physician and applied to several schools in the United States without success. He subsequently went to Ontario, Canada, where as previously mentioned, a large community of African Americans existed. Augusta entered Trinity College of Medicine of the University of Toronto, graduating in 1860[37] as the first African American graduate from a Canadian medical school. He worked at Toronto City Hospital from 1860 to 1863.[17] In March 1863, he wrote from Canada requesting to sit for the examination as surgeon with the United States Colored Troops and was subsequently commissioned Surgeon of Colored Troops[38] in the Union Army in April 1863. Augusta was the first African American to receive a commission as major in the Medical Department of the Union Army. Most of his service was detached from his regiment, and he served in Washington, D.C.; Baltimore, Maryland; and North Carolina and Georgia. At the end of the war, he received a brevet promotion to lieutenant colonel making him the highest ranking African American in the Union Army for several decades. In 1866, when Howard Medical College was opened in Washington, D.C., he was the only African American on the faculty. He stayed on the faculty until 1877 when he entered private practice in Washington, D.C. Augusta died in Washington in 1890.

When John Rapier, Jr., was graduated from the Iowa College of Physicians and Surgeons in Keokuk, Iowa, in 1863,[39] he was the first African American to be graduated in medicine west of the Mississippi River. Rapier's father, John Sr., had been born a slave, and on obtaining his freedom, moved to Canada where the young Rapier was born. Rapier returned to the United States as an adult to find a place to live. He first attended Michigan Medical College for one year but apparently left because of faculty hostility towards him. He spent his second year at the Iowa College of Physicians and Surgeons in Keokuk, Iowa, being graduated in 1863. In 1864 he obtained an appointment as an acting assistant surgeon in the United States Colored Troops. His subsequent life is not chronicled.

The year 1864 marked the graduation of Benjamin A. Boseman and, surprisingly, an African American woman, Rebecca Lee. Benjamin A. Boseman was graduated from the Medical School of Maine in 1864.[22] Boseman was freeborn in New York City, grew up in Troy, New York, and in 1857 was apprenticed locally before attending the Medical School of Maine. In August 1864, he received an appointment as an acting assistant surgeon in the Department of the South[40] and spent the rest of 1864 and 1865 in Hilton Head, South Carolina. He opened a medical practice in South Carolina after the war and subsequently entered politics. In 1868 he was part of the Reconstruction Legislature of that state, serving until 1873 in the state House of Representatives.[41] He became the legislature's member of the board of regents of the South Carolina Lunatic Asylum in 1869, and in 1873 he became the first African American postmaster of the city of

Charleston, South Carolina, serving in that position until his death in 1881.[42] He was complimentary of Democratic Governor Wade Hampton but did not support his re-election in 1878.

Rebecca Lee was born in 1833 and was graduated from the New England Female Medical College[43] in Boston in 1864.[44] Lee was the first African American woman to obtain a medical degree in the United States.[10, 14] Born in Delaware, she was raised by an aunt in Philadelphia and trained as a nurse in Boston in 1852. In 1865, after medical graduation and the fall of Richmond, she went to Richmond where she worked with the freed slaves of that city. In 1867 she married Dr. Arthur Crumpler and moved back to Boston, where she practiced medicine as Dr. Rebecca Lee Crumpler, concentrating on nutrition and preventive medicine. In 1883 she published a work called *Book of Medical Discourses* on the medical care of women and children.[45] She died in 1895. There is a plaque on the house where she practiced, and the house is included in the African American History Tour in Boston.

Charles Burleigh Purvis arrived on the scene as the war was ending. He was born in 1842. Purvis attended Oberlin College in the early 1860s and was graduated from the Medical Department of Western Reserve College, now Case-Western Reserve University in Cleveland, Ohio, in the spring of 1865[46] after completing the required three years of classes. Purvis entered the Union Army in June 1865 and was assigned to Freedmen's Hospital in Washington, D.C. In 1869 Purvis joined the faculty at Howard Medical College and spent the next 54 years of his life with that institution. He was also on the medical staff at Howard Hospital and at times was Chief of Surgery. Purvis died in Washington in 1930.

Alpheus W. Tucker also was graduated in 1865[47] from the Iowa College of Physicians and Surgeons in Keokuk, Iowa. Tucker is known to have attended Oberlin College from 1861 to 1863 but little else is known except that he served as an acting assistant surgeon with the Union Army. In the late 1860s he was in practice in Washington, D.C., and his death was reported in the *Transactions of the American Medical Association*, but the only supporting details were the date and fact of his medical school graduation.

Anderson Ruffin Abbott received his medical degree from the Toronto School of Medicine, Toronto, Ontario, Canada, in 1867.[48] Abbott was Canadian by birth, born in Buxton, Ontario, in 1837. He attended Oberlin College in Ohio and then returned to Toronto, where he served an apprenticeship with Dr. Alexander Augusta. He was licensed to practice medicine in 1861 by the College of Physicians and Surgeons of Ontario, the state medical society. He then began classes at Trinity College, University of Toronto, but had not yet been graduated when he obtained an appointment as acting assistant surgeon with the United States Colored Troops and moved to the United States, where he was assigned to Freedmen's Hospital in

Washington, D.C. In 1866 he returned to Canada and resumed his medical studies. He obtained his medical degree from the Toronto School of Medicine in 1867. Abbott had developed an interest in forensic medicine and was appointed Coroner of Kent County, Ontario, in 1874. He died in December 1913.

These men (and one woman) certainly have the highest medical credentials and are the best documented of the African American physicians, but nevertheless significant details of their life's journey have been lost for many of them. Two other groups of African American physicians are even less well-documented. One group contains those men who have been reported as having been graduated from a medical school, but no such graduation has been confirmed. The second group is men for whom no medical school graduation has been attributed, although some of these men had attended medical school for a period of time. Less educational detail is known but their sacrifices and courage were still considerable.

Chapter 5

Possible Medical School Graduates

There were several men who were believed to have received diplomas, but unfortunately the medical schools traditionally associated with them have no record of their graduation, and often no record of their attendance (Table 3).[9, 10] Oral tradition, unfortunately, is difficult to document. For one individual, two different schools were listed by two different authors, but neither school has a record of attendance or graduation.[9, 18] Two of the men had documented attendance at a medical school for at least one year. Certainly many students moved from school to school for training and many, often due to economic circumstances, simply went into practice without obtaining a diploma. One individual served as a contract surgeon with the Union Army, so his graduation might be presumed since most of the other contract surgeons were medical graduates. In any event, none of these men were found on the lists of graduates from any of the schools known to have awarded diplomas to African Americans. It is possible that graduation was at one of the schools for which the records of graduation cannot be found. It is also possible that attendance was at a school not yet identified as graduating African Americans in that era.

William Miller Dutton attended one year of classes at the Medical School of Maine but did not graduate.[22] No school of graduation has been identified for him and nothing else is known of his history except that he was a resident of New York City.

John H. Fleet was reported to be a graduate of the "old medical school on 10th and E Street" in Washington, D.C.[9, 10] That was the location of the

Table 3: Presumed Medical Graduates, No School Identified

Graduate	Known Affiliation
Dutton, William Miller	Medical School of Maine – 1 yr
Fleet, John H.	
McDonough, David K.	
Powell, Jr., William B.	
Snowden, Isaac H.	Harvard Medical School – part of 1 yr Medical Department of Dartmouth College – 1 yr

National Medical College, later known as George Washington University, but they have no record of attendance or graduation for Fleet.[31] Georgetown, the only other medical school open in the city at that time, also has no record of his attendance.[49] Fleet had been a music teacher in Georgetown prior to entering medicine and ultimately gave up medicine to return to music. He died in 1861. His house in Washington is currently included in the city's cultural tour. To date no medical school attendance or graduation has been confirmed.

David K. McDonough was a slave selected to settle an argument on whether "Negroes possess such innate mental capacity as makes him susceptible to a degree of mental cultivation."[9] He was sent to Lafayette College and then, at his own request, to medical school. His medical preceptor was Dr. John K. Rodgers, who was on the faculty at Columbia University in New York City. Divergent reports have him attending either Columbia University[9] or New York University,[18] but both schools have reported no record of either attendance or graduation of a David K. McDonough.[50, 51] He later joined the staff of the Eye and Ear Infirmary in New York, and was successful. The first private hospital for African Americans in New York was named for him, but the source gives no more details of his life.[9]

William B. Powell, Jr. was a young man about whom little is known. It is known that he was from New York City where his father had a medical practice. Sources state that he served with the Union Army, and as he is not in the official rosters, it is assumed that he served as an acting assistant surgeon. Published letters from his father state that the son was serving in the Union Army in July 1863.

Isaac H. Snowden, who was originally from Boston, was one of the individuals dismissed from Harvard Medical School in 1850.[10] He reapplied to Harvard in 1853 but was rejected. He then matriculated at the Medical Department of Dartmouth College[27] for one session but did not graduate. Where he went from there is not known. There is no record of graduation for him from any of the schools known to have awarded diplomas to African Americans. Prior to his medical school attendance he had been very active in abolition circles in Boston, working as a printer while living on Southac Street in Boston. His admission to Harvard had been sponsored by the American Colonization Society, and he had agreed to emigrate to Liberia after receiving a medical diploma, so there is a possibility that he left the United States.[29] He may have obtained a medical degree from one of sectarian schools for which no records are currently available.

This group of African American men is the most enigmatic. One strives to hear the unspoken, hidden, and lost details. It appears likely that most of these men were medical graduates. The loss of detailed records for so many medical schools of the nineteenth century which are now extinct causes a good deal of frustration in documenting these men.

Chapter 6

Physicians Without Degrees

A number of men who practiced medicine are not known to have received a medical degree (Table 4), and several of these clearly entered medical practice through apprenticeship alone. As previously stated, this was the prevalent route for the majority of physicians early in the nineteenth century and remained the predominant one for African Americans. By mid-century, the majority of white physicians had attended medical school, and a high percentage of those in practice had received degrees prior to beginning practice. Several of these African American physicians had attended medical school but no record has been found of degrees having been obtained. It is probable that the majority of African American physicians by mid-century still attained this status by apprenticeship alone, even though so few names have surfaced. It must be remembered that much of the available data was retained by oral tradition, so misinterpretation of dates and schools is possible.

William Wells Brown[9, 10] was born in 1816, the son of a slave mother and a white physician father. His owner was apparently his father's brother, and he may have been sold at an early age.[17] He was taught to read and write as a child and escaped to the North at age eighteen, becoming part of the abolition movement. Brown wrote and published a fascinating book called *Narrative of William W. Brown, a Fugitive Slave*, on his experiences as a slave. He was very active in abolitionist activities and lectured widely throughout the North.[20] In 1853 he published *Clotel* based on Sally Hemings and Thomas Jefferson, possibly the first novel published by an African American in the United States. He

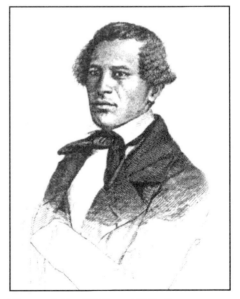

Figure 4. Dr. William Wells Brown
Dr. Brown had been born a slave and practiced medicine learned by apprenticeship. He wrote and published a book about his early life. *Used by permission of the Ohio Historical Society, Columbus, Ohio.*

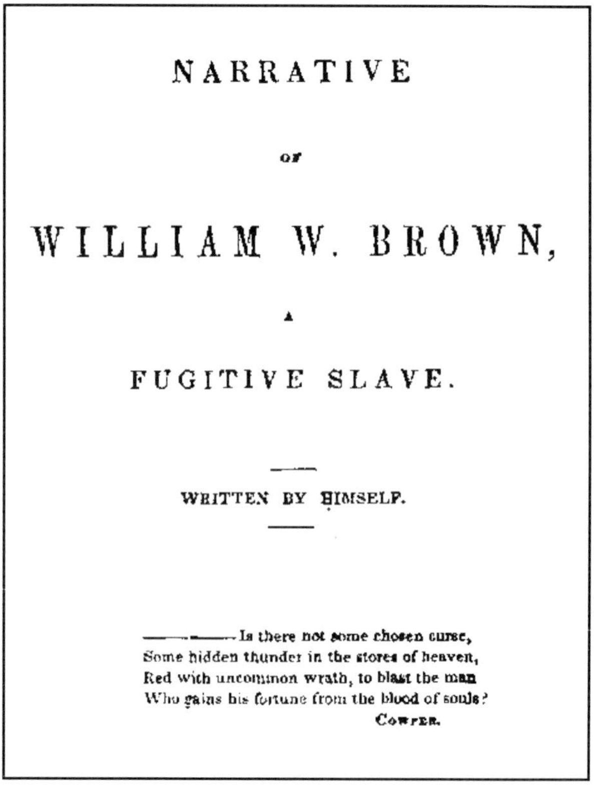

NARRATIVE

OF

WILLIAM W. BROWN,

A

FUGITIVE SLAVE.

WRITTEN BY HIMSELF.

——————— Is there not some chosen curse,
Some hidden thunder in the stores of heaven,
Red with uncommon wrath, to blast the man
Who gains his fortune from the blood of souls?
COWPER.

Figure 5. Title Page of the book by William Wells Brown
Dr. Brown wrote and published this moving description of his early life as a slave and a run-away. *Used by permission of the Ohio Historical Society, Columbus, Ohio.*

Table 4: No Known Degree

Name	School Attended, if any
Brown, William Wells	
Crumpler, Arthur	
Delany, Martin Robison	Harvard Medical School – 1 Yr
Harris, Joseph Dennis	Medical Department of Western Reserve College – 1 Yr
Powell, Sr., William B.	
Reynolds, John P.	
Still, James	
Wells, Lewis G.	Washington Medical College – 1 Yr

traveled widely, including a trip to England. His return to Boston was complicated because the Fugitive Slave Law put him at risk, so his freedom was purchased by friends so that he could return to the United States. Brown then became interested in medicine and attended private medical lectures but not medical school. In 1864 he opened a successful practice in Boston, Massachusetts, as an eclectic physician. He continued to write, publishing several books on history over the next several years. He died in 1884 in Chelsea, Massachusetts, and is buried in Cambridge.

Little is known about Arthur Crumpler. The history of Dr. Rebecca Lee states that they were married in 1867 and moved from Richmond, Virginia, to Boston, Massachusetts. Crumpler's background and training are not discussed in the accounts about Lee. It is presumed that he learned medicine by apprenticeship since he does not appear on any listing of graduates. The accounts of Rebecca Lee Crumpler that detail her life and practice give no details concerning Arthur Crumpler.

Martin Robison Delany is the most illustrious in this group.[9, 52] Delany was freeborn in 1812 in Charleston, Virginia (now West Virginia), and his family moved to Chambersburg, Pennsylvania, when he was ten. At age nineteen, he moved to Pittsburgh, Pennsylvania, and became active and well-known in abolitionist circles. While in Pittsburgh, he published a newspaper called *Whisperer*. Delany became interested in medicine as a career but did not succeed in obtaining admission to a medical school. He then worked with the noted African American publisher and abolitionist, Frederick Douglass, on the *North Star* in Philadelphia. During this time he resumed his interest in medicine and, with further preceptorship, again attempted entry to medical school. Finally, Delany succeeded in being admitted to Harvard Medical School in 1850 at age 38, along with Daniel Laing, Jr. and Isaac H. Snowden. After

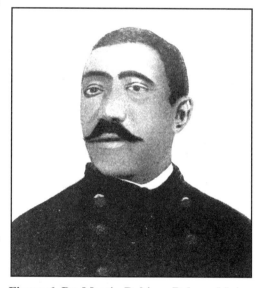

Figure 6. Dr. Martin Robison Delany, Major of Infantry, United States Colored Troops
Dr. Delany attended Harvard Medical School for one year but did not graduate. He practiced medicine and dentistry, having learned both by apprenticeship. His commission as a line officer related to his abolitionist activities.
Used by permission of Source Prints & Photographs/Moorland-Spingarn Research Center, Howard University, Washington, D.C.

being asked to leave Harvard, Delany established a medical practice based on his previous apprenticeship and his limited formal training. He also resumed his abolitionist activities and became involved with colonization, although this was unpopular with the majority of African Americans at the time. As previously mentioned, he and Dr. David Peck organized a settlement in Nicaragua in 1855. This met local resistance, including from the U.S. Navy which is said to have fired on the settlement, and the colony failed. It should be noted that there were many other plans and attempts for colonization but, except for the establishment of Liberia in West Africa, they all shared the same fate. Even the history of Liberia is not a story of success, as more recent accounts have documented.

Delany returned to the United States without Peck and organized an expedition to explore the Niger River in Africa in 1859. His 1861 scientific report on the expedition was well received. Portions of his report and many other anti-slavery papers and lectures are widely quoted.[20] By the time of his return to the United States, the Civil War had begun. He campaigned for a corps of African Americans in the Union Army, led by African American officers. Several early attempts were unsuccessful. After the Emancipation Proclamation in 1863, the decision was made to recruit African Americans as soldiers but only with European American officers. Delany then actively worked as a recruiter for Massachusetts and Rhode Island. He sought a meeting with President Lincoln, and finally in March 1865, Delany obtained a commission as Major of Infantry in the 104th Infantry Regiment, United States Colored Troops with the specific goal of raising a regiment to be officered by African Americans. He was thus the first African American to become a major in a combat unit, although he saw no action. Esther Hill Hawks noted his presence in South Carolina, actively recruiting for his regiment.[53] The war ended before this goal could be accomplished, however, and no new regiments were formed.

After the war, Delany served for some time in South Carolina as an Assistant Sub-Commissioner in the Reconstruction Government. He remained in South Carolina after leaving Federal service, where he apparently supported the candidacy of Wade Hampton for governor in 1876. Hampton's election was a disaster for African Americans because of the rapid return of all-white dominance in the state, and a disappointed Delany apparently spent more time in Central America before returning to Boston. Little was heard from or about him after this and he dropped from prominence. He died in 1885.

Joseph Dennis Harris was from either Virginia or North Carolina. His early life is unknown but he was well-educated. He was interested in abolition and appears to have favored colonization, writing a book promoting emigration to Haiti in 1860. He subsequently developed an interest in medicine and attended classes for one year, 1863-1864, at the

Medical Department of Western Reserve College in Cleveland, Ohio, but was not graduated from there. No record has been found of any subsequent graduation. In July 1864, he was reported to be in Portsmouth, Virginia, and was called doctor. In June he had received an appointment as an acting assistant surgeon with the Union Army. By late 1865 he was in charge of Howard Grove Hospital for the Freedmen's Bureau in Portsmouth. After the war he stayed in Virginia, became active in politics, and in 1869 was defeated as candidate for lieutenant governor of that state.

William B. Powell, Sr., has become known only incidentally.[20] In the search for his son who served with the Union Army, letters were found that were written by the senior Powell and published at that time. It is not known whether his practice was established on the basis of apprenticeship only, or if he had attended some medical school. Because of his having a son old enough to be a physician serving in the army, and the fact that the first known African American received a medical degree in the United States in 1847, it is unlikely that he is a medical graduate because of his presumed age. It is known that he was in successful medical practice in New York City. He reported that his home was threatened and sacked during the draft riots of 1863. He also stated that his eldest son, William B. Powell, Jr., was serving with the Union Army at that time.

John P. Reynolds[9] was self-taught, having been initially trained in "Indian medicine," a non-traditional form of folk medicine. He gradually moved to more conventional medicine and styled himself as an eclectic physician. Reynolds practiced in Zanesville, Ohio, and in Vincennes, Indiana.

James Still[9, 10] was freeborn in 1812 in Burlington County, New Jersey, and grew up with an interest in medicine. He began by reading books and then preparing medicines for neighbors. He continued to read extensively, although he never had a formal apprenticeship or a medical license. Nevertheless, Dr. Still developed a successful practice with both white and African American patients. He practiced for over fifty years, and he wrote an autobiography called *Early Recollections and Life of James Still* which reported some of his favorite cases. Still died in 1872.

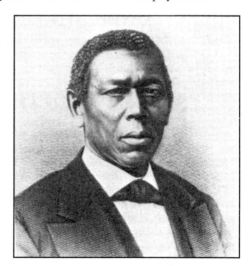

Figure 7. Dr. James Still
Dr. Still learned medicine by apprenticeship and enjoyed a prosperous practice. *Used by permission of the New York Public Library, Schomberg Collection.*

Lewis G. Wells[9] attended Washington Medical College in Baltimore, Maryland, for one year but left after a disagreement with the faculty. The details of the disagreement are not stated, and no record of subsequent graduation from any school has been found. Wells is the second African American known to have attended a Southern medical school in the antebellum years. He subsequently practiced medicine in Baltimore and had a successful career as a physician and a practical phrenologist. He was also an ordained minister of the gospel in the Methodist Church. He died of cholera.

These fascinating stories must be only a small fraction of the stories available "somewhere." If, as Morais contends, the majority of African American physicians learned by apprenticeship only, why are more of them not known and remembered in history? The next portion of this work will present those African American men who heeded the call of freedom and are known to have served with the Union Army during the Civil War.

Chapter 7

Union Army Physicians

The first African American regiments in the United States Army were originally organized as state militia units, and the first regiments to see action were the Louisiana Native Guard in the fall of 1862.[54, 55] These units initially had been organized as the *Corps d'Afrique* of the Louisiana Militia for the Confederate Army but had never been outside of Louisiana. They were designed as combat units and had African American officers as well. After Louisiana was occupied by the Union Army, these units joined the Union Army and later became part of the United States Colored Troops. The 1st South Carolina Infantry (African Descent) was organized by Major General David Hunter in the summer of 1862 and was composed of freed slaves from South Carolina. The unit was not official until January 1863, but they were in combat in November 1862.[54, 55] This unit became the 33rd Infantry Regiment, United States Colored Troops. The 1st Kansas Colored Infantry, later the 79th Infantry Regiment, United State Colored Troops,[55] was organized by Major General James H. Lane, who was the military commander of the region. This unit saw action in October 1862 but was not officially organized until January 1863.[54] President Lincoln had authorized the military to use persons of African descent for any purpose, but apparently had not intended this to mean combat. They were not officially approved for combat service until the issuance of the Emancipation Proclamation on January 1, 1863.

Initially, Secretary of War Edwin M. Stanton decreed that all officers in the African American units would be white. The original Louisiana units had all African American officers and the Kansas regiment had several. Most of these officers were replaced by white officers. Later the policy was softened to allow African American surgeons and chaplains when available. The Bureau of Colored Troops was created by General Order No. 143,[56] May 1863, and all but a few of the existing state regiments were then designated United States Colored Troops. Some units, such as the 54th Massachusetts Infantry (the first regiment of colored troops authorized after January 1, 1863, though not the first activated) were, for political reasons, allowed to keep state designations. By the end of the war, at least 111 African Americans had served as officers,[54] and ninety of these officers were in combat units. Seventy-six African American officers served with the previously-mentioned Louisiana Colored Regiments. Ultimately, some 180,000 African American men served in the Union Army.

Physicians were one group of officers needed by these units. An official United States Army Board was created to examine physicians to serve as medical officers with the United States Colored Troops. Although these troops were officially considered state volunteer units, the examination of candidates for appointment as medical officers was federally controlled. The initial choices were white physicians, but many white doctors did not want to serve with colored troops, so there were difficulties obtaining adequate numbers of medical officers for these regiments. Parenthetically, it should be mentioned that a chronic shortage of commissioned medical officers existed army-wide and this shortage was supplemented by the appointment of contract surgeons. Some men serving as hospital stewards were, in fact, commissioned as medical officers for the Colored Troops.[57] It is possible that not all of these were trained physicians, although many hospital stewards had some medical school attendance or were physicians who had not yet passed, or could not pass, the rigorous medical examination required for army physicians. It is also possible that the examination for qualification of this group was made less strenuous, but this is unlikely since no inference has been documented. A number of African Americans had been graduated from United States and Canadian medical schools by this time,[17] and a group of these men were ultimately selected to serve with the United States Colored Troops.

Commissioned medical officers at the regimental level consisted of two grades. Each regiment had one surgeon with the rank of major, and one or more assistant surgeons with the rank of captain or first lieutenant. A hospital had a Surgeon-in-Charge with other surgeons and assistant surgeons below him. When additional physicians were needed, the Surgeon-in-Charge could hire temporary help called contract surgeons, and they held the official title acting assistant surgeon. Contract surgeons could be hired to work in any army activity but were most commonly used in the general hospitals. Many appointments were short term, often for just one battle, although by 1863 appointments were sought for a minimum of three months.[58]

Official listings may not even include all contract surgeons. An official list exists for all regimental and staff surgeons and assistant surgeons who were commissioned officers, but no complete register exists for acting assistant surgeons. Due to this, any tabulation of the actual number of contract surgeons must be regarded as an approximation. It should be emphasized that contract surgeons were not considered active-duty military personnel but only civilians, as is the case today. At that time, many of the contract surgeons wore a uniform, often with the rank insignia of captain or first lieutenant (see the photograph of Dr. Abbott on page 36), although this was not a requirement. The official salary for a surgeon was $163 per month. An assistant surgeon received $112.33 per month while a contract surgeon received slightly less, usually $100 per month, and, of course, no potential for retirement with paid pension. Inflation increased these amounts as the war progressed.

At least three African Americans were commissioned medical officers during the Civil War. The remaining nine African American physicians identified as serving with the army and the United States Colored Troops were contract surgeons. They were appointed, not commissioned, as acting assistant surgeons. This, then, leads to the final two chapters and the discussions of African American physicians in the Union Army as a group. Some of the material included in these chapters is repeated from previous chapters in detail to present a more complete picture of the serving officers.

Chapter 8

Commissioned Officers

The first African American to receive a commission as surgeon in the Army was Alexander Thomas Augusta (Table 5).[9, 17, 36, 59] Augusta was freeborn in Norfolk, Virginia, on March 8, 1825, and became interested in medicine. To finance his training, he journeyed to California in search of gold. When he was unable to gain admittance to an American college of medicine because of his race, Augusta moved to Ontario, Canada. After serving an apprenticeship, he was admitted to Trinity College of Medicine, University of Toronto, Ontario, Canada. In 1860[37] he was graduated and worked at Toronto City Hospital. After the activation of the United States Colored Troops, he applied for and was granted a commission. When Augusta appeared before the Examining Board in March 1863, with the appropriate invitation in hand, the Board was uncertain regarding what action to take when it noted that he was "of African descent." The Board requested direction from the Surgeon General's Office "since no other medical officers of this descent or color had been commissioned."[60] It was decided to allow the examination and a commission if justified by its results.

On April 4, 1863, Augusta was commissioned surgeon and ultimately assigned to the 7th Infantry Regiment, United States

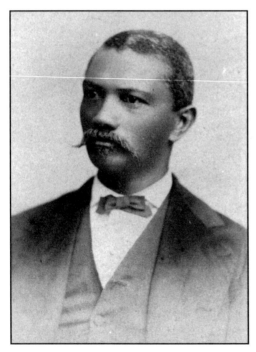

Figure 8. Alexander Thomas Augusta, M.D., Surgeon, United States Colored Troops
Dr. Augusta was graduated from University of Toronto College of Medicine, Toronto, Ontario, Canada, in 1860. He was the first African American member of a medical faculty in the United States. *Used by permission of Source Prints & Photographs/ Moorland-Spingarn Research Center, Howard University, Washington, D.C.*

Table 5. Commissioned Medical Officers

Surgeon	Unit
Augusta, Alexander Thomas	7th USCT
	Trinity College, University of Toronto
McCord, David O.	66th Illinois Infantry &
	63rd USCT
	Medical College of Ohio
	Assistant Surgeon
DeGrasse, John Van Surly	35th USCT
	Medical School of Maine

Colored Troops.[38] Thus he became the first African American to be commissioned as a major in the United States Army, although some writers have given this distinction to others, notably Martin Delany who did not receive his commission until March 1865. Augusta was initially assigned to a Camp for Colored Persons in the Military District of Washington. Two white assistant surgeons at the camp felt that they could not work under a colored officer since no other white officer was doing so. Subsequently Surgeon Augusta was reassigned[17] to examine recruits at Birney Barracks in Baltimore, while retaining his rank within the 7th U. S. Colored Troops. The assistant surgeon of the 7th USCT renewed his complaint concerning working as a subordinate to an African American surgeon in the spring of 1864 because he wanted Augusta removed from the regiment so that he might obtain the promotion. Although the army never officially responded to this complaint, Augusta spent the rest of his time on detached duty in Beaufort, South Carolina, and Savannah, Georgia.[60] He remained on the roster of the regiment throughout the war.

When war commissions were terminated in November 1866, Augusta continued to work as a contract surgeon for the army until March 1867. In July 1867, he received a retroactive promotion to Brevet Lieutenant Colonel for "faithful and meritorious service," dating from March 13, 1865, until he was discharged from the army in 1866. A brevet promotion was temporary, usually for meritorious service. Augusta was the only African American to achieve this rank until the end of the nineteenth century.[9]

There is an interesting anecdote concerning the acceptance of African Americans in Washington, D.C. The *Congressional Globe* (the official record of Congress) dated February 9, 1864, discusses an incident where Surgeon Augusta, in his army uniform, was refused passage on the city railway because of his race.[61] Senator Henry Wilson from Massachusetts was so upset that he achieved passage of a law stating that blacks should have equal access to the street railway.[62] This story was picked up by the

Richmond Examiner, a Confederate newspaper in Richmond, Virginia.[63] An article dated April 6, 1864, entitled "Negro Equality in the North" gave a verbatim account of the *Congressional Globe* report and adds the comment: "These extracts, in our judgment, show clearly and conclusively 'the mission of the war.'"

When Howard Medical College was founded in 1868, Augusta was the only African American member of the original faculty.[9, 17, 36, 59] He was named Demonstrator of Anatomy, doing dissections and showing anatomic details to the students. He had several subsequent appointments at Howard Medical College and became Chairman of the Department of Anatomy. In 1877 Augusta left the medical school but continued to practice in Washington, D.C., and he was among the first African Americans to apply for membership in the Medical Society of the District of Columbia.[64] Unfortunately, he was denied membership in the society and in the American Medical Association. Augusta continued to practice in Washington until his death in December 1890. He is buried in Arlington National Cemetery.

The second African American to receive a commission as Surgeon was David O. McCord. McCord was freeborn in Kentucky in 1830 and his family moved to Illinois in 1833. He apprenticed in medicine and then was graduated from the Medical College of Ohio in 1854.[30] After graduation he opened a medical practice in the small town of York, Illinois. Special Order No. 114, Vicksburg, Mississippi, dated December 1, 1863,[65] states that Surgeon D. O. McCord of the 9th Louisiana Volunteers, later renamed the 63rd United States Colored Infantry, had been appointed Medical Director and Inspector of Freedmen. Surgeon McCord[38] is described in his orders as "of African descent." The appointment was only for the regiments raised by Colonel John Eaton, the newly-created Superintendent of Freedmen for the region. These troops were to guard the laborers of Freedmen camps and plantations in the Department of Tennessee and the State of Arkansas. McCord's given name was not stated in the orders or in the official register of regimental officers, even though a federal regulation specifically stated that either the first or the second name of every man mustered must be spelled out completely in the regimental muster rolls.

In March 1863, McCord wrote to the Surgeon General of the Army[66] asserting that he was on active duty and had been commissioned as such on November 11, 1862, with date of rank specified as from May 9, 1862. He explained that he was the second assistant surgeon of the 66th Illinois Infantry, originally known as "Birge's Western Sharpshooters," which had been organized under the special patronage of Major General John Fremont. On arrival he was detached to act as surgeon for the Cassele Engineer Corps (colored troops). On January 13, 1863, McCord was re-assigned to the Contraband Hospital where he was serving when he wrote the letter to the Surgeon General. It should be noted that Birge's Western Sharpshooters was not, and never had been, a colored unit—thus McCord was serving in a white unit. It also should be noted he was serving in the army at a time when no Colored Troops had yet been authorized by the President. McCord's letter is given further credence by a letter from the Surgeon General's Office to the Commissioner of Pensions.[66] The second letter, dated February 3, 1893, states that David O. McCord served as assistant surgeon with the 66th Illinois Infantry and as surgeon with the 63rd Infantry Regiment, United States Colored Troops. McCord is, therefore, the first African American physician to receive a commission as an assistant surgeon in the Union Army during the Civil War.

Following the war, McCord returned to practice medicine in Illinois until his death in 1874 from "systemic congestion." At the time of his death, he was a member of the Illinois chapter of the American Medical Association, and his obituary is reported in the *Transactions of the American Medical Association*. He was said to have "an enviable reputation in his profession," and he was described as a man "of decided ability, great energy, and industry."[30]

John Van Surly DeGrasse is the third man known to have received a commission in the Union Army. DeGrasse was the second African American to be graduated from an American college of medicine. He was graduated in 1849 from the Medical School of Maine,[22] affiliated with Bowdoin College, in Brunswick, Maine. Following graduation, he traveled to Paris and ultimately became Assistant Dresser (performing tasks similar to an assistant resident today, assisting in surgery and caring for the patient) for the famous French surgeon, Alfred A. L. M. Velpeau.[9, 10] DeGrasse returned to the United States after two years in Paris and initially practiced in New York. He moved to Boston, Massachusetts, where he was very successful and even became a member of the Massachusetts Medical Society. After the war began and regiments of Colored Troops were formed, he applied for a medical commission. He was commissioned in September 1863 as an assistant surgeon[38] with the 35th Infantry Regiment, United States Colored Troops, as confirmed in

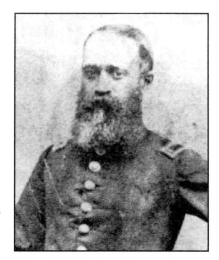

Figure 9. John Van Surly DeGrasse, M.D., Assistant Surgeon, United States Colored Troops
Dr. DeGrasse was the second African American to receive a medical degree in the United States when he graduated from Medical College of Maine, Brunswick, Maine, in 1849. *Used by permission of the New York Public Library, Schomberg Collection.*

his compiled military records.[60] His presence with the 35th USCT is documented by Dr. Esther Hill Hawks, who met him in South Carolina.[53] After the war DeGrasse returned to Boston and resumed his practice. Governor John A. Andrew of Massachusetts presented DeGrasse with a ceremonial surgeon's sword to show the appreciation of the people of Massachusetts for his service in the Civil War.[17]

It is necessary to include Martin Robison Delany in this chapter since he also was given a commission in the Union Army as a major. However, this commission was not in the Medical Department but in the infantry.[9, 17] Delany's checkered career is described earlier. It is often stated that he was the first African American to receive a commission as major in the Union Army, but again, the commissions of both Augusta and McCord pre-date Delany's commission by one and one-half years to two years.

Chapter 9

Contract Surgeons

In addition to the commissioned officers, nine other African Americans are reported to have served with the Union Army (Table 6).[17] The biographical sketches of many of these men state an appointment as acting surgeon or acting assistant surgeon. The title of "acting surgeon" did not officially exist, so they must have been appointed as acting assistant surgeons. Others are said to have served at the Freedmen's Hospital but no specifics are given regarding rank or status. Since the majority of medical officers working at the general hospitals were acting assistant surgeons, one must assume this title for such men. As stated earlier, these men were contract surgeons. For simplicity of discussion, these men will be presented here in alphabetical order rather that by chronology.

Table 6. Contract Surgeons (Acting Assistant Surgeons)

Surgeon	School
Abbott, Anderson Ruffin	Toronto School of Medicine
Boseman, Benjamin A.	Medical School of Maine
Creed, Cortlandt van Rensselaer	Yale University Medical School
Ellis, William B.	Medical Department of Dartmouth College
Harris, Joseph Dennis*	Medical Department of Western Reserve College
Powell, Jr., William B.	Unknown
Purvis, Charles Burleigh	Medical Department of Western Reserve College
Rapier, Jr., John	Iowa College of Physicians & Surgeons
Tucker, Alpheus W.	Iowa College of Physicians & Surgeons

*Attended 1 year only, no known degree

Anderson Ruffin Abbott was born in Canada and grew up in Ontario, Canada. He attended Oberlin College in Ohio, after which he moved to Toronto. Abbott spent four years apprenticed to Dr. Alexander T. Augusta and then began medical school at the University of Toronto. In 1861,

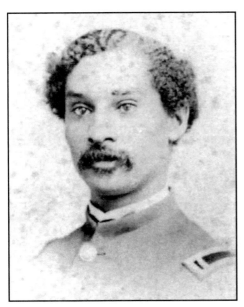

apparently based on his apprenticeship, he received a medical license from the College of Physicians and Surgeons of Ontario.[37, 48] This is the official name of the medical society of the province of Ontario, and this organization had the authority to grant medical licensure. In 1863

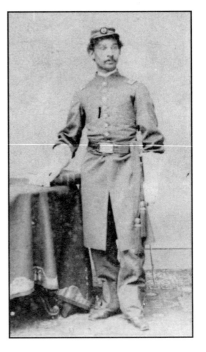

Figure 10. Anderson Ruffin Abbott, M.D., Acting Assistant Surgeon, United States Colored Troops
Dr. Abbott was licensed by the College of Physicians and Surgeons of Ontario in 1861. After the Civil War he returned to Canada and was graduated from the Toronto College of Medicine, Toronto, Ontario, Canada, in 1867. a: Portrait. b: Full-length picture in the uniform of the United States Colored Troops. *Used by permission of the Ontario Reference Library – A. R. Abbott Papers, Toronto, Ontario, Canada.*

when Dr. Augusta entered the Union Army, Abbott also applied for military service. At that time he stated he would be receiving his Bachelor of Medicine degree from the University of Toronto in the spring of 1863. In September 1863, Abbott was appointed acting assistant surgeon[67] and was assigned to the Freedmen's Hospital in Washington, D.C. He also worked in several hospitals serving Colored Troops and former slaves in Washington. In 1866 Abbott returned to Canada, resuming his practice and training. He received a Bachelor of Medicine degree in 1867 from the Toronto School of Medicine,[37] a school affiliated with the University of Toronto. For reasons unknown, the afore-mentioned graduation from the University had not happened. In 1869 Abbott became a member of the College of Physicians and Surgeons of Ontario and served, subsequently, as the President of the

Kent County Medical Society, Kent County, Ontario, Canada. In 1874 he was appointed Coroner of Kent County. He died in December 1913.

Benjamin A. Boseman was born in New York City and grew up in Troy, New York, subsequently apprenticing with a physician in that city.[41] He was graduated from the Medical School of Maine in 1864 and in August of that year received an appointment as an acting assistant surgeon in the Department of the South of the Union Army,[40] serving in Hilton Head, South Carolina. After the war, he established a medical practice in South Carolina and became active in politics in that state, becoming a member of the 1868 Reconstruction Legislature and serving in the state House of Representatives until 1873. In 1869 he was appointed to the board of the state lunatic asylum. Boseman became the first African American postmaster of the city of Charleston in 1873 and served in that position until his death in 1881.[42]

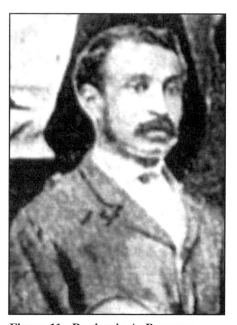

Figure 11. Benjamin A. Boseman, M.D., Acting Assistant Surgeon, United States Colored Troops
Dr. Boseman was graduated from the Medical School of Maine in 1864. He remained in South Carolina at the end of the war and became active in politics. He served in the 1868 Reconstruction Legislature and became Postmaster of the City of Charleston in 1873. *Used by permission of Emily E. Vaughn.*

Cortlandt van Rensselaer Creed was the first African American to be graduated from Yale University.[33] Creed was freeborn in New Haven, Connecticut, where his father worked at the faculty club of Yale University and became an admirer of another Yale graduate, financier Cortlandt van Rensselaer, for whom he named his son. Creed received his medical degree in 1857 and practiced in New Haven, Connecticut. With the onset of war, he advocated the use of African American troops, as did many northern African American abolitionists. Once the United States Colored Troops were created, he applied for a commission as a medical officer. In 1863 Creed received an appointment as acting assistant surgeon with the 30th Connecticut Volunteers (Colored Troops).[32] At the end of the war, he resumed his practice in Connecticut and developed a significant reputation in forensic medicine. In 1876 he was appointed Justice of the Peace in Connecticut.

William B. Ellis was an 1858 graduate of the Medical Department of Dartmouth College.[27] He also served as a physician in the army.[17] Few details of his life are known but he did receive an appointment as an acting assistant surgeon in March 1864.[40]

Joseph Dennis Harris was from either Virginia or North Carolina.[68] The details of his early life are largely unknown, although at some point he received a good education. As with many educated African Americans of the time, he was interested in abolition and apparently favored colonization. In 1860 he published a book called *A Summer on the Border of the Caribbean Sea*, as Mr. J. Dennis Harris, extolling the merits of emigration to Haiti.[68] The development of his interest in medicine is not known, but he did attend medical school for the 1863-1864 term at the Medical Department of Western Reserve College, Cleveland, Ohio.[46] Although no medical school graduation has been documented for him, however, he was in Portsmouth, Virginia, in the summer of 1864 and was being called "doctor." A report in *The Christian Recorder* in July 1864[69] identifies Harris as a U. S. surgeon and indicates that he was very knowledgeable, although his exact duty is not stated. He is known to have received an appointment as an acting assistant surgeon in June 1864.[40]

Dr. Ira Russell describes Dr. Harris in his U. S. Sanitary Commission Reports,[70] as "an extremely intelligent colored gentleman from Cleveland, Ohio." Harris was in charge of Howard Grove Hospital which was operated by the Freedmen's Bureau in Portsmouth, Virginia, in late 1865. He is said to have seen "considerable service and is well-respected." Dr. Russell's comments indicate that Harris had seen and cared for African American soldiers over a significant period of time. Certainly Harris is described as being very knowledgeable about diseases among African American soldiers. His presence as Surgeon-in-Charge of Howard Grove Hospital is also mentioned in a December 23, 1865, article in *The Christian Recorder*.[71] Little is know about the activities of Harris after the war except that he apparently stayed in Virginia and became active in politics. In 1869 he was a candidate for lieutenant governor.[72] He was defeated by J. F. Wells by a vote of 120,068 to 99,600.

William B. Powell, Jr.,[9, 17] has no known medical school education and no particulars of appointment are available. Like Dr. Tucker, he is assumed to have been an acting assistant surgeon. The classic book, *The Negro's Civil War*, quotes two letters by a Dr. William B. Powell from New York.[20] Although in the majority of instances biographical information is given about the people quoted, in this instance he is simply identified as "Dr. William B. Powell, a Negro physician." In one of these letters, he describes his experiences as a victim of property damage in the race riots in New York City, and in another letter, Dr. Powell states that his eldest son was serving as "a surgeon with the United States Army." The son is the Dr. Powell of interest here, and this is further confirmation of his service. Since all but one of the other African American physicians known to have served with the Union Army were medical graduates, the assumption is made that Dr. William B. Powell, the younger, was probably also a medical school graduate, although it is agreed that he may have had some medical education but not a diploma, as in the case of Dr. Harris. Powell possibly was also apprenticed by his father.

Charles Burleigh Purvis was born on April 14, 1842. He attended Oberlin College and then graduated from the Medical Department of Western Reserve College, now Case-Western Reserve University,[46] in the spring of 1865, just as the war was ending. He obtained an appointment with the army as an acting assistant surgeon in June 1865,[40, 73, 74] after the end of the hostilities. Purvis was assigned to the Freedmen's Hospital in Washington, D.C., his contract stating that he would be paid $113.85 per month.[75] In 1869 Purvis joined Howard University as the second African American member of the faculty of the College of Medicine, initially teaching Materia Medica. Purvis spent the next fifty-four years affiliated with the school and held many different positions. He was on the medical staff of Howard Hospital and at times served as the Chief of Surgery. One published anecdote is a rumor that he was not reappointed Chief of Surgery at Howard Hospital in 1901, primarily because his wife was a white woman from Connecticut. This was not, at that time, socially acceptable in the local community. Despite such obstacles, Purvis was very important to the survival of the Howard Medical College in its early years.[73]

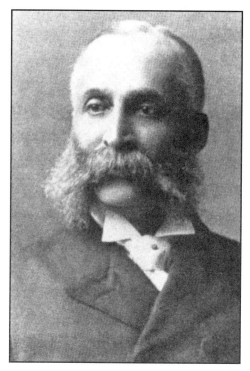

Figure 12. Charles Burleigh Purvis, M.D., Acting Assistant Surgeon, United States Colored Troops
Dr. Purvis was graduated from Medical Department of Western Reserve College, now Case-Western Reserve University, Cleveland, Ohio, in 1865. His subsequent presence on the faculty of Howard Medical College was crucial to its continued survival. *Used by permission of Source Prints & Photographs/Moorland-Spingarn Research Center, Howard University, Washington, D.C.*

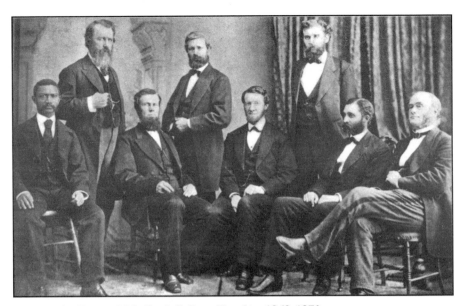

Figure 13. Howard Medical College Faculty, 1869-1870

The individuals are (front row, l-r) A.T. Augusta, G.S. Palmer, R. Reyburn, C.B. Purvis, P.H. Strong; (back row, l-r) S.L. Loomis, O.O. Howard, J.T. Johnson. Drs. Augusta and Purvis were the only African American members of the faculty at that time. *Used by permission of the Moorland-Spingarn Research Center, Howard University Archives, Washington, D.C.*

John Rapier, Jr., was the son of a slave who had obtained his freedom and emigrated from the United States to Canada, living in the settlement of freemen and freed slaves in Buxton, Ontario. Rapier began his life in Canada but traveled extensively as an adult to find a place to live. He subsequently came to the United States, first to Minnesota and then to Ohio. He attended medical school for one year at the Michigan Medical College and then went to the Iowa College of Physicians and Surgeons in Keokuk, Iowa.[17, 39] In 1863 he became the first African American to be graduated from a medical school west of the Mississippi River. After graduation he sought, and in June 1864, obtained an appointment as an acting assistant surgeon,[40] serving at Freedmen's Hospital in Washington, D.C. His subsequent life is not chronicled. Verification of his graduation from the medical school mentioned is not possible because the location of any remaining archives has not been found.

Little is known about Alpheus W. Tucker[17] except that he served with the Union Army as an acting assistant surgeon.[40] He is said to have been graduated from the Iowa College of Physicians and Surgeons in 1865.[47] He is mentioned in the History of the Medical Society of the District of Columbia as having applied for membership in June 1869, at the same time as Dr. Augusta. It is further stated that his credentials were found appropriate but he was not elected.[64] Tucker's death was reported in the *Transactions of the American Medical Association.*

This, then, lists all of the African Americans known to have served as acting assistant surgeons in the Union Army. These nine men served in a different capacity but, along with the three commissioned officers, comprise the twelve men known to have served with the Union Army.

Chapter 10

Conclusion

The story of these early African Americans in medicine is a proud but neglected one, an important but little-known chapter in the history of medical education and medicine in the United States. As stated, it is difficult to find details, and it is almost certain that this work constitutes only a portion of the history that can and should be written on this subject. It is likely, as stated by Morais, that more apprentice-trained physicians were in practice than medical school graduates but, while emphasizing a traditional mode of practice comparable to that of the country as a whole, the medical graduates are easier to find since some independent documentation exists. Reliance on oral history for dates and places is a disadvantage. Hopefully, this new information age will allow greater access to any records that exist and stimulate more individuals to look into their family histories.

It is indeed impressive that these men, during this time, achieved medical school attendance and graduation. It is even more impressive that they would achieve commissions in the Medical Department of the Union Army, where the standard of practice was much higher than in the community at large. Their willingness to serve certainly demonstrates a high level of caring and concern.

The chapter on physicians in the Union Army details the men who are known to have served. The author's search for information for this manuscript added four new men to the oft-cited list of African American surgeons in the army, increasing the known number by fifty percent. It is assumed that there are others who could be added to this list. These men took the adventure of a formal medical education even further and put themselves and their lives on the line for freedom. Their efforts need to be remembered. As with the other parts of this history, the known information is often fragmentary.

This work is not a complete record of the events of those times. Additions can and should be made to this list, and missing information will appear. Missing here means "not in the public eye and difficult to find," not necessarily "non-existent." Hopefully, future work will more fully document this epic journey.

Bibliography

1. Norwood WF. *Medical Education in the United States before the Civil War*. Philadelphia: University of Pennsylvania Press; 1944.

2. Packard FR. *History of Medicine in the United States*. New York: Paul Hoeber, Inc.; 1931.

3. Waite FC. American Sectarian Medical Colleges Before the Civil War. *Bull Hist Med*. 1946;19:148-166.

4. Shryock RH. Women in American Medicine. *J. A. M. W. A.* 1950;5(9):371-279.

5. Spiegel AD, Suskind PA. Mary Edwards Walker, M.D.: A Feminist Physician a Century Ahead of Her Time. *J Commun Health*. 1996;21(3):211-235.

6. Sanes S. Elizabeth Blackwell: Her First Medical Publication. *Bull Hist Med*. 1944;16:83-88.

7. Blake JB. Women in Medicine in Ante-bellum America. *Bull Hist Med*. 1965;36(2):99-123.

8. Yandell DW. Presidential Address. *Transactions of the American Medical Association*. 1872;23:85-103.

9. Farmer HE. An Account of the Earliest Colored Gentlemen in Medical Science in the United States. *Bull Hist Med*. 1940;8:559-618.

10. Cobb WM. The Black American in Medicine. *J Nat Med Assoc*. 1981;73(Supp):1185-1242.

11. Bousfield MO. An Account of Physicians of Color in the United States. *Bull Hist Med*. 1945;XVII:61-84.

12. Mansfield CM. African Americans in Radiation Oncology. In: Gagliardi RA, Wilson JF, eds. *A History of the Radiological Sciences: Radiation Oncology*. Reston, VA: Radiology Centennial, Inc.; 1996.

13. Watson WH. *Against the Odds: Blacks in the Profession of Medicine in the United States*. New Brunswick, NJ: Transaction Publishers; 1999.

14. Epps Jr CD, Johnson DG, Vaughn AL. *African-American Medical Pioneers*. Baltimore: William & Wilkins; 1994.

15. Segars JH. Prologue: Black Soldiers in Gray? In: Barrow CK, Segars JH, Rosenburg RB, eds. *Black Confederates*. Gretna, LA: Pelican Publishing Company; 1995:1-6.

16. Duffy J. *The Sanitarians: A History of American Public Health*. Chicago: University of Illinois Press; 1992.

17. Morais HM. *The History of the Negro in Medicine*. New York: Publishers Company, Inc.; 1969.

18. Delany MR. *The Condition, Elevation, Emigration, and Destiny of the Colored People of the United States, Politically Considered*. Philadelphia: Martin R. Delany; 1852.

19. Records of Attendance and Graduation, Glasgow University Medical College. Located at: University of Glasgow, Glasgow, Scotland.

20. McPherson JM. *The Negro's Civil War*. First Vintage Civil War Library Edition ed. New York: Vintage Books, Random House; 1965.

21. Records of Medical Graduation, Rush Medical College. Located at: Rush Medical College, Chicago, IL.

22. Records of Medical Graduation, Maine Medical College. Located at: Bowdoin College, Brunswick, ME.

23. Waite FC. *The First Medical College in Vermont, Castleton, 1818-1862*. Montpellier, VT: Vermont Historical Society; 1949.

24. Parsons WS, Drew MA. *The African Meeting House: A Sourcebook*. Boston, MA: The Museum of Afro American History.

25. Larson KC. *Bound for the Promised Land. Harriet Tubman, Portrait of an American Hero*. New York: Ballantine Books; 2004.

26. McPherson JM. *The Battle Cry of Freedom: The Civil War Era*. New York, NY: Ballantine Books; 1989.

27. Records of Medical Graduation, Dartmouth Medical College. Located at: Dartmouth University, Hanover, NH.

28. Walsh MR. *"Doctors Wanted: No Women Need Apply." Sexual Barriers in the Medical Profession 1835-1975*. Binghamton, NY: Yale University Press; 1975.

29. Menard L. *The Metaphysical Club*. Boston, MA: Farrar, Straus & Giroux; 2001.

30. Chew SC. Report of American Medical Necrology. *Transactions of the American Medical Association*. 1875;26:451-478.

31. Records of Medical Graduation and Attendance, National Medical College. Located at: George Washington University, Washington, DC.

32. Yale University. *The First African American Graduate From Yale University in 1857*. New Haven, CT: Yale University; Feb 8, 2001.

33. Records of Graduation, School of Medicine, Yale University. Located at: Yale University, New Haven, CT.

34. New Orleans Library. *African Americans in New Orleans*. New Orleans, LA 2002.

35. Records of Graduates of the Western College of Homeopathy, Dittrick Medical History Center. Located at: Case-Western Reserve University, Cleveland, Ohio.

36. Newby MD. Augusta, Alexander Thomas. *American National Biography*. Vol 1. New York: Oxford University Press; 1999:752-754.

37. Records of Medical Graduation, Trinity College. Located at: University of Toronto, Toronto, Ontario, Canada.

38. Hambrecht FT, Ed. *Roster of Regimental Surgeons and Assistant Surgeons in the U. S. Army Medical Department during the Civil War*. Gaithersburg, MD: Olde Soldier Books, Inc.; 1989.

39. Newby JD. Thomas/Rapier Family Archives Web Site. *Buxton Historical Site*. 8/1/1998. Available at: www.ciaccess.com/~jdnewby.

40. Index to Contract Surgeons, Entry 45; Records of Surgeon General's Office, Record Group 112; National Archives Building, Washington, DC.

41. Foner E. *Freedom's Lawmakers: A Directory of Black Officeholders during Reconstruction*. New York, NY: Oxford University Press; 1993.

42. Miller RM, Andrus AT. *Witness to History: Charleston's Old Exchange and Provost Dungeon.* Orangeburg, SC: Sandlapper Publishing Inc; 1986.

43. Waite FC. *History of the New England Female Medical College, 1848-1874.* Boston: Boston University School of Medicine; 1950.

44. Records of Graduation, New England Female Medical College. Located at: Boston University, Boston, MA.

45. Potter J, Clayton C. *African-American Firsts.* Elizabethtown, NJ: Pinto Press; 1994.

46. Records of Graduation, Medical Department of Western Reserve College. Located at: Case-Western Reserve University, Cleveland, OH.

47. Genealogical Records: *Directory of Deceased American Physicians 1804-1929.* Family Tree Maker's Family Tree, Broderbund, The Learning Company, 1999.

48. Newby MD. *Anderson Ruffin Abbott: first Afro-Canadian Doctor.* Markham, Ontario, Canada: Associated Medical Services: Fitzhenry & Whiteside; 1998.

49. Records of Attendance and Graduation, Georgetown University Medical School. Located at: Georgetown University, Washington, DC.

50. Records of Attendance and Graduation, Medical College of New York. Located at: New York University, New York, NY.

51. Records of Attendance and Graduation, College of Physicians and Surgeons. Located at: Columbia University, New York, NY.

52. Cobb WM. Martin Robison Delany. *J Nat Med Assoc.* 1952;44(3):232-238.

53. Schwartz G, ed. *A Woman Doctor's Civil War: Esther Hill Hawks' Diary.* Columbia, SC: University of South Carolina Press; 1984.

54. Hollandsworth Jr. JG. *The Louisiana Native Guards: The Black Military Experience During the Civil War.* Baton Rouge, LA: Louisiana State University Press; 1995.

55. Weidman B. Preserving the Legacy of the United States Colored Troops. National Archives and Records Administration [Web Site]. 2/20/1998. Available at: www.nara.gov/education/teaching/usct/usctart.html.

56. United States War Department. *The War of the Rebellion: A Compilation of the Official Records of the Union and Confederate Armies.* Vol III. Washington, DC: Government Printing Office; 1880-1901.

57. Medical News, Army Medical Intelligence. *American Medical Times*; April 14, 1864.

58. Tripler CS. Report of Surgeon Charles S. Tripler, Medical Director of the Army of the Potomac, of the Operations of the Medical Department of That Army from August 12,1861, to Mar 17, 1862. In: United States War Department, ed. *The War of the Rebellion: A Compilation of the Official Records of the Union and Confederate Armies.* Vol V. Washington, DC: Government Printing Office; 1880-1901.

59. Cobb WM. Alexander Thomas Augusta. *J Nat Med Assoc.* 1952;44(4):327-329.

60. Compiled Service Records, Records of the Adjutant General's Office, Record Group 94; National Archives Building, Washington, DC.

61. *Congressional Globe*, 38th Congress, First Session, Feb 9, 1864; pp.553-555, Washington, DC.

62. Berlin I, Reidy JP, Rowland LS, eds. *Freedom: A Documentary History of Emancipation, 1861-1867. Series II: The Black Military Experience.* Cambridge: Cambridge University Press; 1982.

63. Negro Equality in the North. *Richmond Examiner.* April 6, 1864.

64. Lamb DS, Franzini CW, Cook GW, Holden RT, Eliot L. *History of the Medical Society of the District of Columbia.* Washington, DC: Medical Society of the District of Columbia; 1909.

65. Medical News. Army Medical Intelligence. *American Medical Times.* Jan 9, 1864.

66. Pension Papers, David O. McCord; Entry 561, Records of the Adjutant General's Office, Records Group 94; National Archives Building, Washington, DC.

67. Newby MD. Abbott, Anderson Ruffin. *American National Biography.* Vol 1. New York: Oxford University Press; 1999:15-16.

68. Harris JD. *A Summer on the Border of the Caribbean Sea*, with an introduction by George William Curtis, 1860, A. P. Burdick, Publisher. In: Bell HH, ed. *Black Separatism and the Caribbean 1860.* Ann Arbor, MI: University of Michigan Press; 1970.

69. A Letter from Virginia by LOOK IN, July 2, 1864. *The Christian Recorder*, July 9, 1864.

70. Russell I. Series 1. Medical Committee Archives, 1861-1865. Located at: United States Sanitary Commission Records, Reel 3, Frame 5, Rare Books and Manuscripts Division, New York Public Library, New York, NY.

71. A Letter from Richmond, Nov 7, 1865, by W. D. S. *The Christian Recorder*, Dec. 23, 1865.

72. *The Negro in Virginia.* Washington, DC: Works Progress Administration, Government Printing Office; 1940.

73. Cobb WM. Charles Burleigh Purvis. *J Nat Med Assoc.* 1953;45(1):79-82.

74. Newby MD. Purvis, Charles Burleigh. *American National Biography.* Vol 17. New York: Oxford University Press; 1999:947-948.

75. Personal Papers, Charles Purvis; Entry 561, Records of the Adjutant General's Office, Record Group 94; National Archives Building, Washington, DC.

About the Author

Robert G. Slawson, MD, FACR, is a retired physician who spent 28 years as faculty member of the Department of Radiation Oncology at the University of Maryland School of Medicine in Baltimore, Maryland, after serving eight years with the United States Army Medical Corps. Since his retirement he has focused his interests in history and medical history to concentrate on medicine of the Civil War era. He has given lectures and written several papers on this subject. He is a Master Docent at the National Museum of Civil War Medicine in Frederick, Maryland.

Index

1st Kansas Colored Infantry 27

1st South Carolina Infantry (African Descent) 27

7th Infantry Regiment, United States Colored Troops 30, 31

9th Louisiana Volunteers 32

30th Connecticut Volunteers (Colored Troops) 37

33rd Infantry Regiment, United States Colored Troops 27

35th Infantry Regiment, United States Colored Troops 33

54th and 55th Massachusetts Infantry Regiments 13

54th Massachusetts Infantry 27

63rd Infantry Regiment, United States Colored Troops 32, 33

66th Illinois Infantry 14, 32, 33

79th Infantry Regiment, United State Colored Troops 27

104th Infantry Regiment, United States Colored Troops 24

A

A Summer on the Border of the Caribbean Sea 38

Abbott, Anderson Ruffin 10, 17, 28, 35, 36

abolition 8, 9, 12, 13, 15, 20, 21, 23, 24, 38

acting assistant surgeon 15, 16, 17, 20, 25, 28, 35, 37, 38, 39, 40

African Free School 9

allopathy 1

American College of Medicine 10, 13

American Colonization Society 14, 20

American Medical Association 14, 17, 32, 33, 41

Andrew, John A. 13, 34

apprentice 2, 3, 5, 7, 12, 13, 14, 16, 17, 21, 23, 24, 25, 26, 30, 32, 36, 35, 39, 42

Arkansas 14, 32

Arlington National Cemetery 32

assistant surgeons 28, 29, 31, 35, 41

Augusta, Alexander Thomas 10, 15, 16, 17, 30, 31, 32, 34, 35, 36, 40, 41

B

Baltimore, Maryland 14, 16, 26, 31

Beaufort, South Carolina 31

Bias, James Joshua Gould 10, 12

Birge's Western Sharpshooters 32

Birney Barracks 31

Book of Medical Discourses 17

Boseman, Benjamin A. 10, 16, 35, 37

Boston, Massachusetts 4, 10, 11, 13, 17, 20, 23, 24, 33, 34

botanic medicine 1

Bowdoin College 11, 33

Bowers, Catherine 13

Boylston, Zabdiel 4

British Columbia 15

Brown, William Wells 21, 22

Brunswick, Maine 10, 11, 33

Buchan's *Domestic Medicine* 5, 33

Bureau of Colored Troops 27

Burlington County, New Jersey 25
Buxton, Ontario 17, 40

C

Caesar 4, 5
California 30
Cambridge, Massachusetts 23
Camp for Colored Persons 31
Canada 12, 15, 16, 17, 30, 35, 36, 37, 40
Case-Western Reserve University 17, 39
Cassele Engineer Corps (colored troops) 32
Castleton, Vermont 10, 11
Castleton Medical College 10, 11
Celebration, Annual Crispus Attucks 13
Chambersburg, Pennsylvania 23
Charleston, South Carolina 5, 17
Charleston, West Virginia 23
Chase, Salmon P. 13
Chelsea, Massachusetts 23
Chicago, Illinois 9, 10
Cincinnati, Ohio 10, 14
City Gazette and Daily Advertiser 5
Cleveland, Ohio 10, 15, 17, 25, 38
Clotel 21
College of Physicians and Surgeons of Ontario 17, 36
colonization 14, 20, 24, 38
Colored Orphan Asylum 9
Columbia University 20
commission 11, 14, 16, 24, 30, 31, 32, 33, 34, 37, 38, 42
Congressional Globe 31, 32
Contraband Hospital 32
contract surgeons iii, 19, 28, 29, 31, 35
Corps d'Afrique 27

Creed, Cortlandt van Rensselaer 10, 14, 15, 35, 37
Crumpler, Arthur 17, 22, 23
Crumpler, Rebecca Lee 17, 23

D

DeGrasse, John Van Surly 10, 11, 31, 33
Delany, Martin Robison 11, 14, 22, 23, 24, 31, 34
Delaware 17
Department of Tennessee 14, 32
Derham, James 4, 5
Detroit, Michigan 15
Douglass, Frederick 23
Dunbar, Charles 10, 13
Dutton, William Miller 19

E

Early Recollections and Life of James Still 25
Eaton, John 32
eclectic 1, 12, 13, 23, 25
Eclectic Medical College of Philadelphia 10, 12
Ellis, William B. 10, 15, 35, 38
Emancipation Proclamation 24, 27
England 5, 14, 17, 23
Examining Board 30
Eye and Ear Infirmary 20

F

Fleet, John H. 19, 20
folk medicines 2, 25
freeborn 4, 9, 12, 14, 15, 16, 23, 25, 30, 32, 37
Freedmen's Bureau 25, 38

Freedmen's hospital 14, 17, 35, 36, 39, 40
Fremont, John 32
Fugitive Slave Law 23

G

George Washington University 14, 20
Georgia 16, 31
Gibbons, Quinton 12

H

Hahneman, Samuel C. F. 1
Haiti 24, 38
Hampton, Wade 17, 24
Hanover, New Hampshire 10, 13
Harbert, Samuel 13
Harris, Joseph Dennis 22, 24, 35, 38
Harvard Medical School 14, 19, 20, 22, 23
Hawks, Esther Hill 24, 34
Hemings, Sally 21
heroic medicine 1
Hilton Head, South Carolina 16, 37
Holmes, Oliver Wendell 14
homeopathy 1, 15
hospital stewards 28
Howard Grove Hospital 25, 38
Howard Hospital 17, 39
Howard Medical College 16, 17, 32, 39, 40
Hunt, Harriot Kesia 14

I

inoculation 4, 5
Iowa College of Physicians and Surgeons 10, 16, 17, 35, 40

J

Jefferson, Thomas 21
Jenner, Edward 5

K

Kansas 27
Kearsley, John, Jr. 5
Kent County Medical Society 37
Keokuk, Iowa 10, 16, 17, 40

L

Lafayette College 20
Laing, Daniel, Jr. 10, 13, 14, 23
Lane, James H. 27
Leach, Robert B. 10, 15
Lee, Rebecca 10, 16, 17, 23
Liberia 20, 24
lieutenant governor 25, 38
Louisiana 6, 15, 27, 32
Louisiana Colored Regiments 27
Louisiana Native Guard 27

M

Massachusetts 4, 5, 11, 13, 23, 24, 27, 31, 33, 34
Massachusetts Bar 13
Massachusetts Magazine 5
Massachusetts Medical Society 11, 33
Mather, Cotton 4
McCord, David O. 10, 14, 31, 32, 33, 34
McDonough, David K. 19, 20
Medical College of Ohio 10, 31, 32
Medical Department of Dartmouth College 10, 13, 15, 19, 35, 37, 38
Medical Department of Western Reserve College 10, 17, 22, 25, 35, 38, 39

medical examination 28

Medical School of Maine 10, 11, 16, 19, 31, 33, 35, 37

Medical School of Yale University 14

Medical Society of the District of Columbia 32

Michigan Medical College 16, 40

Minnesota 40

Morgan, John 2

N

Narrative of William W. Brown, a Fugitive Slave 21

National Medical College 10, 14, 20

New Amsterdam 4

New England Female Medical College 10, 17

New Haven, Connecticut 10, 14, 37

New Orleans, Louisiana 15

New York City 9

New York State Medical Society 12

Nicaragua 11, 24

Niger River 24

Norfolk, Virginia 15, 30

North Carolina 16, 24, 38

North Star 23

O

Oberlin College 17, 35, 39

officers iii, vii, 24, 27, 28, 29, 30, 32, 35, 41

Ohio 14, 15, 17, 25, 32, 35, 38, 40

Onesimis 4

Ontario, Canada 15, 16, 17, 30, 35, 37

P

Peck, David 9, 10, 11, 24

Pennsylvania Gazette 5

Philadelphia, Pennsylvania 2, 5, 10, 11, 12, 13, 15, 17, 23

Philadelphia College of Medicine 2

phrenologist 12, 26

Pittsburgh, Pennsylvania 23

Portsmouth, Virginia 25, 38

Powell, William B., Jr. 19, 20, 25, 35, 38, 39

Powell, William B., Sr. 22, 25, 38

Primus 4, 5

Purvis, Charles Burleigh 10, 17, 35, 39

R

Rapier, John, Jr. 10, 16, 35, 40

rattlesnake bite 5

Ray, Peter William 10, 11, 12

Reconstruction Legislature 16, 37

Republican National Convention 15

Reynolds, John P. 22, 25

Richmond, Virginia 17, 23, 32

Richmond Examiner 32

Rock, John Sweat 10, 12, 13

Rodgers, John K. 20

Roudanez, Louis Charles 10, 14, 15

Royal Society 4, 5

Rush Medical College 9, 10

Russell, Ira 38

S

Salem, New Jersey 12

Santomé, Lucas 4

Savannah, Georgia 31

sectarian 1, 2, 3, 8, 15, 20

Sharpe, Jacob 12

Simon 4, 5

slaves vii, 4, 5, 15, 16, 17, 20, 21, 23, 27, 36, 39

smallpox 4, 5

Smith, James McCune 9, 10

Snowden, Isaac H. 19, 20, 23

South Carolina 5, 11, 16, 17, 24, 27, 31, 34, 37

South Carolina Lunatic Asylum 16

Stanton, Edwin M. 27

Still, James 22, 25

Sumner, Charles 13

Superintendent of Freedmen 32

Supreme Court 13

surgeon 5, 11, 14, 15, 16, 17, 19, 20, 25, 28, 30, 31, 32, 33, 34, 35, 37, 38, 39, 40

Surgeon-in-Charge 28, 38

T

Taylor, William Henry 10, 14

Thomson, Samuel 1

Thomsonian medicine 1

Toronto, Ontario, Canada 10, 16, 17, 18, 30, 35, 36

Toronto City Hospital 16, 30

Toronto School of Medicine 10, 17, 18, 36

Transactions of the Royal Philosophical Society 5

Trinity College 16, 17, 30, 31

Troy, New York 16, 37

Tubman, Harriet 13

Tucker, Alpheus W. 10, 17, 35, 40, 41

U

Underground Railroad 12

United States Colored Troops 11, 13, 14, 16, 17, 24, 27, 28, 29, 30, 31, 32, 33, 36, 37

University of Glasgow 9, 10

University of Paris 15

University of Pennsylvania College of Medicine 2

University of Toronto 10, 16, 17, 30, 31, 35, 36

V

vaccination 5

Velpeau, Alfred A. L. M. 33

Vincennes, Indiana 25

Virginia 15, 23, 24, 25, 30, 32, 38

W

Washington, D.C. 10, 14, 15, 16, 17, 19, 20, 26, 31, 32, 36, 39, 40

Washington Medical College 14, 22, 26

Watson, Samuel C. 10, 14, 15

Wells, J. F. 38

Wells, Lewis G. 22, 26

West Virginia 23

Western College of Homeopathy 10, 15

Whisperer 23

White, Thomas Joiner 10, 11

Wilson, Henry 31

Windsor, Connecticut 5

women vii, 2, 3, 17

Woodward, John 4

Y

Yale University 10, 14, 37, 35, 37

York, Illinois 14, 32

Z

Zanesville, Ohio 25